ALIVE AT 65...
GREATER
AT 80!

by Sandra Mortensen, PT

Balance
Flexibility
Strength

How to make it easy
Where to begin

This book will help you learn a simple
fitness plan for life. It is designed
to build a bridge from work into
retirement and the road beyond.

www.BalanceFlexibilityStrength.com

ALIVE AT 65... GREATER AT 80!

by Sandra Mortensen, PT

EXERCISE DISCLAIMER

All informational content is for educational purposes only. Always consult a qualified medical professional before beginning any exercise program. The information contained herein is not a substitute for professional medical advice, diagnosis, or treatment. Consult your physician or other qualified health provider with any questions regarding any medical condition. Use of this information is solely at your own risk.

- Sandra Mortensen, PT

AUTHOR'S NOTE

Are You the Audience for This Book?

This book is for people who have realized they need to move or move more for better health and quality of life but don't know how to begin and don't like the word "exercise."

This book is for someone who already "works out" or goes to the gym but is getting older and looking for simplicity in fitness routines or what to do when there isn't a gym or equipment available.

This book is for the person who has picked up numerous exercise books but found they are hundreds of pages long, and the exercises are too difficult, or there are too many exercises.

My focus: Create easy-to-learn movement routines for balance, flexibility, and strength.

Turn the page and get started if this appeals to you!

TABLE OF CONTENTS

Smile! Breathe! Begin!

CHAPTER 1

WHY DID I WRITE THIS BOOK?

I am a retired physical therapist living in the heart of ski country, Summit County, Colorado. I was passionate about my profession. I was passionate about helping people overcome pain, injury, or surgery. I was passionate about assisting people to improve the quality of their physical lives and the ability to keep moving. I am now sharing that passion through this book.

In the last years of working full time in my sports medicine and pain management physical therapy practice, I noticed a common thread in the exercises I gave my clients. Their problems varied: joint and muscular issues or pain in general. All benefited in their recovery from similar components in rehabilitation routines.

I also noticed some of my clients, primarily in their 50s, 60s, and 70s, having generally diminished strength, flexibility, and balance, which interfered with their quality of life. Loss of muscle mass, decreased joint mobility, and reduced sense of where we are in space increase as we age. It was upsetting to hear their complaints of fading energy and endurance, loss of strength, and general stiffness, now compounded by their injuries and pain. Today, there is overwhelming evidence that staying active reduces loss of **Balance, Flexibility, and Strength** into older age.

The rehabilitation routines I taught my clients included general balance, flexibility, and strengthening. The result was not just recovery from the injury, but also improvement in their overall health, sense of well-being, and quality of life. They now had routines they could easily continue for the rest of their lives.

Could I motivate my clients to not only work to recover from knee, back, or shoulder surgery or injury but also give them a program they could continue to use for a better quality of life? That answer was "Yes!"

Through this process, I realized I too needed to use the exercise routines for balance, flexibility, and strength for a sense of well-being and continued good quality of life into my older years. As of this writing, I am 80. I wanted to continue skiing, hiking, and traveling, so I would be able to walk, climb stairs, and carry luggage. My friends constantly asked what I was doing to stay fit. I started this program for my clients, tweaking the various routines for each individual's issue. I began doing these routines myself and then shared them with friends. I continue to do them. My friends encouraged me to write his book.

The goal of the routines in this book is not to lose weight. The goal is to be fit and have the balance, flexibility, and strength to move in older age, doing the activities of daily life as well as activities on a bucket list. Also, the goal is to have a decreased fear of falling, fear that increases with age for many.

Along the way, we face challenges to beliefs, habits, and attitudes about "exercise" that may get in our way to beginning or changing a fitness program. I'll talk about overcoming challenges in this book. If your goal is to have the balance, flexibility, and strength to live your life with freedom to move, better health, energy, and a sense of well-being, then continue reading.

My vision is to see motivated women and men with a fitness plan for a better quality of life, using easy routines one can do anywhere; in a bedroom, a hotel room, on a beach, or by a stream, all without equipment.

Do you already have a fitness program in your life, but it may not be working as well as you would like as you move along life's journey? Or are you looking for something new? Have you made changes in your life such that you are no longer going to a gym? Or are you just not motivated to go to a gym but feel it's time to add a fitness routine in your life? Maybe you are retired, exercise very little, and want to start a fitness routine. Or perhaps the word "exercise" just has a negative connotation for you and you don't even want to think about beginning an exercise program.

Where to begin?

It all begins with a decision to bring a balanced, flexible, and strong body along for life's journey as we move into older age. It's a decision that allows you to do all the activities on your bucket list. It's a decision to have more energy for day-to-day activities as well as having a quality, healthy life day to day. We are all unique in where we start. This journey begins with accepting your balance, flexibility, and strength where you are here and now. Then you can make a plan to keep or improve your level of fitness. We all move along on this journey and into our older years in our own unique ways. The key word is "move." As I move into my older years, I want to continue to be able to physically move, so I have a fitness plan. I want to help you to have one too.

Being able to move leads to living well and aging well. Aging well leads to living the life you envision and doing the activities on your bucket list. To do this, we need to keep moving!

Henry Ford said, "Whether you think you can or you think you can't...you are right."

CHAPTER 2

LIVING FIT

A bridge from work into retirement and the road beyond, with energy for living a quality life!

Planning for retirement? Already retired?

Did you make a plan for your retirement? Did you write it down? Save money to retire? Make a bucket list of things to do and places to go in retirement? You may plan to have the money to retire and a bucket list of things to do, but did you include a plan to bring a body along to live the life you dreamed of in retirement? Will you have the energy or level of fitness to live the lifestyle you choose in retirement that you always dreamed of? If you didn't include a plan to bring a fit body along to do all the activities on your retirement bucket list, it doesn't matter how much money or how many bucket list items you have if you have a hard time moving.

I consider a physical fitness plan an integral part of retirement planning. It is never too early or too late to add a fitness element to your life plan or your retirement plan. Studies show that good health and the ability to move are the key drivers of happiness in day-to-day living and in retirement. A regular fitness routine contributes to good health, and being fit contributes to the continued ability to move, creating a quality of life.

As we get older, many develop problems with their bodies, resulting in increased stiffness, joint pain, unsteadiness, or the need for surgery. Even with various infirmities, people who work at being fit improve their quality of life. I can't emphasize enough that **it's never too late to start**. You can bring a body along to do all the activities on your bucket list and improve the quality of your day-to-day life right now.

So, let's begin with two routines to start every day, one to wake up your brain and one for balance.

WAKE UP YOUR BRAIN

Routines to integrate the left and right sides of your brain. Improves balance, vision, mental acuity, and ability to focus.

Cross Crawls

1. Hand to Shoulder

- Stand on both feet.
- Touch left hand to right shoulder and look at left hand.
- Then touch right hand to left shoulder and look at right hand.
- Alternate touching and looking at your shoulders.

5 - 10 repetitions

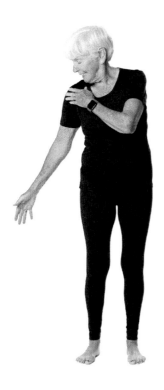
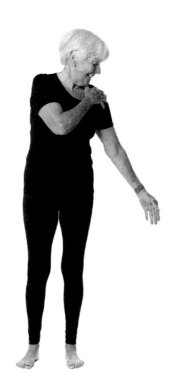

Cross Crawls

2. Hand to Hip

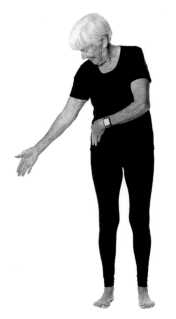

- Stand on both feet.
- Touch left hand to right hip and look at left hand.
- Touch right hand to left hip and look at right hand.
- Alternate touching and looking at your hips.

5 - 10 repetitions

3. Hand to Knees

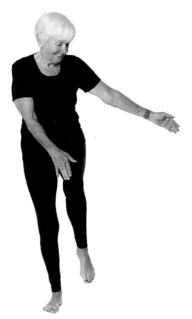

- Stand on right foot.
- Bring left knee up.
- Touch right hand to left knee.
- Look at right hand.
- Alternate touching each knee, looking at the hand and knee touched.

5 - 10 repetitions

What's working: Improved balance, flexibility, and strength, including eye muscles, integrating the left and right sides of your brain, contributing to focus and stability.

Smile! Breathe!

Challenge Your Balance

Why balance? Falling and fear of falling creep up on us as we get older. Falls are close to the number one cause of injury as we get older. Our balance is a component of stability (more on that later). So, wake up your brain, then spend 2-4 minutes on balance to start every day.

Do Your Wake-Up Your Brain Routines Before You Challenge Your Balance!

Balance Challenge

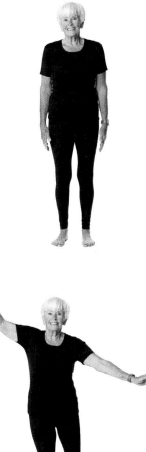

- Stand near a counter or wall in case you need support.
- Alternate balancing on one leg at a time for as long as you can, eyes open, looking straight ahead.

Shoes on is easier, shoes off is harder. Hard or wood floors are easier, carpet is harder.

Use your arms to help you balance or the back of a chair, or touch a wall for assistance if necessary. Toe touch with the opposite foot for occasional assistance if necessary.

2 - 5 repetitions on each leg

Goals:

No chair, counter, wall or toe touch for assistance. Increase the time you can stand on each leg.

I'll make balance more challenging later in the book.

Smile! Breathe!

CHAPTER 3
CHANGE, MOTIVATION, AND CHALLENGES

Or, What Gets in The Way of You Being Fit for Living Your Life!... Or Making Any Life Changes!

Whether beginning a fitness routine or changing the one you have, the operational word is **"change"**. There are many things that contribute to our ability to make changes: our beliefs, our attitudes, our comfort levels, or the voice in our head. To begin, establish a Vision, set specific Goals to achieve that Vision, and then establish Action Plans to achieve your Goals to live your Vision. You took a step by picking up this book. As we get older, we lose muscle mass. This leads to loss of **Balance**, **Flexibility** and **Strength**. Everyone needs a fitness plan, a plan to be able to continue to move along life's journey. The primary question is: What will motivate you to have fitness Goals and a fitness Action Plan to live your Vision? What changes in your beliefs, attitudes, and comfort levels do you need to make to start?

Start with a vision of your life three to five years from now. Where do you want to live? In the city, in the country, in the East, in the West, a larger home, a smaller home, a condo, a senior living community? Do you want one floor or two floors? Do you want outdoor activities available? Museums and libraries? Driving? Not driving? Travel? Write down your answers. Read them out loud. Add to your list as you think of more. Eliminate items as they become irrelevant.

Now focus on the "doing" part of your Vision. What do I want to be doing in the next three to five years? Do I want to be playing tennis, playing golf, walking 1-3 miles a day, continue working, retire, travel, go to the symphony or a play?

Here is a list you may not be thinking about:

- Easily get in and out of bed.
- Get on and off the toilet.
- Get in and out of a bathtub or shower.
- Get up and down from the floor.
- Empty the dishwasher.
- Carry groceries in from the car.
- Put groceries away.
- Get dressed and undressed.

Make your list of what you want to be able to do three to five years from now. Start your list with "I can…"

Here are other things to think about in creating your Vision. How will your life be if you are fit? How will you feel? How will you look? Visualize the level of fitness, **Balance**, **Flexibility**, and **Strength** you will have. Visualize the impact on your self-esteem, your acceptance of your body, and your ability to move easily during your life's activities. Visualize the impact fitness will have not only on you, but also the impact on others in your life if you are able to move and be healthy.

The first step in motivation to start or continue a fitness routine is to have a Vision. Having a vision of how you want to feel and look, gives what you want to do purpose to your fitness plan. Having a fitness plan helps overcome any voices of resistance in your head or from folks around you. This is your journey for living your life.

My fitness vision is to have the **Balance**, **Flexibility**, and **Strength** to travel, ski, and walk on the beach or in the woods.

Step #1:

Write down your life's vision. Share it with friends and family. Read it out loud once in a while. (See the Workbook, Page 13)

In this book, I will focus on the "doing" parts to achieve your Vision: setting Goals and making Action Plans. In other words, Goals with Action Plans to have the **Balance**, **Flexibility,** and **Strength** to live your Vision.

Set Goals that are specific, simple, and achievable in a short amount of time. An example: "I will do some routines four days a week for a minimum of five minutes a day for the next month."

As you move along in this process, delete Goals as they are achieved. Then add new Goals. This is a work in progress, a journey for life.

Step #2:

Make Action Plans to achieve your Goals. Write them down. Action Plans are what you will do, how often you will do it, where you will do it, and how much time you will commit to doing it to achieve your Goals. Once you get started, you may need to make changes to your Action Plans. Don't be hard on yourself. As with Goals, make Action Plans that are specific and achievable. You are looking to be successful. (See the Workbook, Page 13)

Time as a Motivator

Make time a motivator for your success and not a barrier to it. There are several components to time. When do you want to make time for functional balance, functional flexibility, and functional strength routines? Morning, midday, afternoon, or evening? How much time will you spend doing these routines? Choose the time of day and how much time you will spend doing your routine to achieve that goal. Choosing a time of day and the amount of time to work your plan leads to creating a habit. This may be as little as 5-10 minutes in the morning and maybe again in the afternoon. Will you work your Action Plan daily? Three times a week? Make this a part of your plan. Now is not the time to be overly optimistic. Less is better. Start slowly. Write it down. Your action or inaction today influences all your tomorrows.

Environment as a Motivator

Make your environment a motivator for your success and not a barrier to it. Choose a location to do your routines that is pleasing to you. Do you like to stay in the same location or vary that location…bedroom, living room, a grassy park, by a stream, or at a beach? Do you want to be on a carpet or a hard surface? Some of us like other people around who are working out too. This may be in a group setting like a recreation center or just with a workout buddy. Some of us like to be alone: "I don't want anyone to see me doing this." Some of us need to go to a specific place in the house or outside of the home. Some like to wear certain clothes to work out, or no clothes. Some like music. Do you know if you like to work out with music, or no music? If so, what kind of music?

The Voice in Your Head as a Motivator

Make the voice in your head a motivator for your success. Your brain is powerful. Our attitude, beliefs, and the words we use quietly in our head, say out loud, or in writing contribute to success in all areas of our lives. Our words affect our motivation as well as our ability to succeed with our goals and action plans. Talk in a positive, supportive, "can do" voice. It is motivating to have some positive words, affirmations, or mantras to say out loud or read, such as "I can do this." "I have time to do this." "I am capable of doing this." Are you worth it to look better, feel better, have more energy, and be healthier? "YES…I am worth it, and I can DO IT!"

Communication as a Motivator

Have a process to share your Vision, Goals, and Action Plans with friends and/or family, in a journal, in a blog, or on social media. By communicating your Vision and plans, you can elicit support. It helps you stay on task until doing some part of your Action Plan daily becomes a habit. Sharing your Action Plan is an opportunity to release fears or anxieties that keep you from achieving your Goals.

Success as a Motivator

Your fitness is your responsibility. Success doesn't happen overnight. Success comes from working on your Action Plan a little every day. Be patient with yourself. Remember, the #1 supporter, champion, and cheerleader of your plan is YOU! Have the passion, perseverance, and consistency to work your action plans, and you can achieve your goals.

A brief word about success: For me, success means I do something every day for **Balance**, **Flexibility,** or **Strength**. It may be for five minutes, or it may be for an hour. My personal Goal is to establish the habit of moving daily for a minimum of 10 minutes. If it's only for 10 minutes, I focus on Balance and upper or lower body Flexibility. You may choose Balance and Strength routines. What contributes to meeting your Goals?

Do You Want to Make a Change?

The next question: "What concerns you the most about yourself and being able to live your Vision, to want to make a change?" A change to choose to add a fitness routine so you can have the **Balance**, **Flexibility**, and **Strength** for a better quality of life going forward?" It all begins with a decision to bring a strong, flexible, balanced body along for life's journey that allows you to do all the activities on your bucket list and have a good quality of life day to day. We are all unique in where we start. The journey begins with accepting your **Balance**, **Flexibility**, and **Strength** where you are here and now. Then you can make an Action Plan to begin, to keep or to improve your current level of fitness. We all move along on this journey into our older years in our own unique ways.

The Keywords Are:
- I accept where I am now.
- I decide to change and move now!

Write down your answers for your **Vision,** your **Goals**, and your **Action Plans**. Action Plans don't work unless you do. So get to work. Just begin!

CHAPTER 4

WORKBOOK PAGES

Why do I want to develop/maintain/improve my fitness, Balance, Flexibility, and Strength?

It is easier to make an Action Plan, if you know why you are doing this.

What bothers me enough that I want to make a change? Or, what activities do I want to do that I need to be fit to be able to do?

1.

2.

3.

My Vision of being a fit person 3-5 years from now:

How will I feel?

What will I be able to do?

How will being fit will impact my life?

How will my life be different if I am fit?

My Action Plans to achieve my Goals:

How much time a day or a week will I take to make my life changes in my Action Plan?

Where do I want to do my fitness routines? List all the possibilities.

Music? No music? Music on my phone? Computer? Other?

Alone? With a friend? Who? In a group? Where?

My positive affirmations or mantras: Words/phrases/affirmations/mantras I want to hear or tell myself to support my progress.

Ways I will share what I am doing to be more fit.
Examples: I will share My Vision, My Goals, and My Action Plans by calling supporters and friends, using social media, and/or writing in a journal.

I will share my Action Plan with: _____

How? _____

How often? _____

What Balance, Flexibility, and Strength fitness Goals will I make to accomplish my Vision? Do I want weekly, monthly, or quarterly **Goals**?

Each Goal needs an Action Plan.

Suggestions for Action Plans:

- The activity and where will I do this activity?
- How often will I do each activity?
- How much time will I spend each workout period?
- Date I will re-test. (See page 29 for Balance Test.)

You may want to read the rest of this book, then fill out these Goals.

Balance Goal:

Action Plan(s) to achieve this Goal:

Flexibility Goal:

Action Plan(s) to achieve this Goal:

Strength Goal:

Action Plan(s) to achieve this Goal:

CHAPTER 5

WHAT ARE FUNCTIONAL BALANCE, FUNCTIONAL FLEXIBILITY, AND FUNCTIONAL STRENGTH?

Functional: Having an activity, purpose, or task relating to how something works or operates. Designed to be practical and useful rather than attractive.

Functional Balance

Balance is the ability to move away from the mid-line and return without falling down. As we get older, we tend to lose our ability to balance. Studies show that more than 1/3 of older adults fall each year. The number of falls increases with age and are primarily due to loss of **Balance, Flexibility, and Strength**. Falls are the leading cause of injury leading to hospitalization in older adults. Some literature reports that 95% of hip fractures are caused by falls.

We have specialized mechanisms, proprioceptors, that help us keep from losing our balance. Proprioceptors are like little microswitches embedded in muscles, ligaments, tendons, and joints. Proprioceptors can be switched on with movement. Proprioceptors help to tell which muscles to work without us thinking about it so we don't fall down while doing an activity.

Proprioceptors are trainable to improve our ability to not lose our balance, but only if we ask them to do some work every day. Balance routines activate our proprioceptors without us having to think about what to do when the activity involves a need to balance. We can turn them on, make them work, and make them more responsive by challenging them daily with a balance routine. This allows us to improve our ability to recover without falling if we lose our balance. If our balance mechanisms are challenged regularly, we can maintain or improve our ability to balance into older age. The ability to regain balance, not fall, can be improved no matter how young or old we are. Do some balance routines every day!

We do activities that require balance while standing on two feet and while standing on one foot. Standing in place and reaching for an object on the counter, reaching for a forehand shot in tennis, getting something from a high shelf, and returning to standing and not falling down require balance. Balance is more difficult when standing on one foot and even more difficult with an uneven surface. It is also more difficult to move, our upper body while on one foot. Balance requires strength in your core, or trunk, and legs. Balance requires some flexibility.

Your eyes also play a part in your ability to balance. Some exercises incorporate vision, or where you are looking while doing the routine. Balance requires both sides of your brain to be working. (See "Wake Up Your Brain Routines"). I will give you balance tests and exercises to activate your brain and proprioceptors (the microswitches that activate muscles and joints) for better balance.

Functional Flexibility

Functional Flexibility means you have the range of motion or ability to bend and straighten joints enough to do your daily activities, like dressing, getting in and out of a car, or participating in sports. **Functional Flexibility** also means you aren't too stiff to go through the range of motion required to do an activity well or easily.

As we get older, we lose elasticity and plasticity (flexibility) in our tendons and ligaments. If we don't keep moving, muscles and tendons shorten. This causes us to be less flexible unless we ask those joints to keep moving. If we move all our joints through all available range of motion every day, the muscles, tendons, and ligaments have a higher probability of keeping their flexibility. Suppose we don't do this every day. Over time, the decreased elasticity and decreased movement causes the muscles, tendons, and ligaments to get shorter and shorter, losing range of motion and losing their flexibility. This leads to losing the ability to move enough to do the activities we want to do. The result: It is harder to bend over to put on our socks or bend enough to put on our slacks, get in and out of a car, reach the higher shelves in our kitchen, or participate in our favorite sports activity.

How can we improve **Functional Flexibility**? Start by performing a movement with a static stretch. A static stretch is moving to the end range of motion that the joint or joints can accomplish without pain and holding it in that position. **Functional Flexibility** is achieved by adding movement to a static stretch. Stretching with movement, or a dynamic stretch, is more functional and useful in day-to-day activities than a static stretch.

"Static" means "fixed: not moving; motionless." A static stretch is when you move to the end range of motion and hold that position to stretch muscles and ligaments around a joint or joints. A static stretch is a non-functional stretch, meaning your body usually does not know how to incorporate the added length into movement required in a task or sport.

"Dynamic" means "a process characterized by constant change or having a component of activity or movement."

Functional Strength

To have **Functional Strength**, many muscles work together in your arms, legs, and trunk to do a task successfully. Muscles in your body work as a team to do an activity.

An example of strength that may not be functional: Body builders who want to enter competitions to show off their big muscles may not have functional strength. They can show you their big muscles, but what can they actually do with them? Can they easily hit a tennis ball, ski down a ski slope, or play golf or soccer? **Functional Strength** also means you can get up from the floor if you fall down. **Functional Strength** means you can get on and off a toilet or in and out of your car.

Functional Strength means that while you are moving, you have the strength to carry out a task, such as carrying the groceries from the car or participating in a sports activity that requires functional strength, like tennis, skiing, hiking, and carrying a pack or suitcase. **Functional Strength** also means you have the core strength, leg strength, flexibility, and balance to stand on one leg and kick a soccer ball, hit a tennis ball, or put a plate away on a high shelf in the kitchen. Core strength contributes to stability. Stability is a component of being able to move and not fall.

I often see people in a gym sitting on a piece of equipment, kicking up against a resistance bar to strengthen the quadricep muscles in the upper thigh, or lying face down on a machine and bending a knee toward their butt against a resistance bar to strengthen the hamstring muscles (muscles on the back of the thigh). These exercises may increase strength but not functional (usable) strength. Muscles don't work individually or in isolation. Muscles work as a team, some lengthening, some shortening, some getting stronger, while some are letting go, relaxing.

There are many components to **Functional Strength**. For example, to increase **Functional Strength** in your lower extremities, you need to do strengthening routines with your feet or a foot on the ground and not just address individual leg muscles. There needs to be a component of flexibility and balance in order to use the strength in your legs. Also, the quadriceps and hamstring muscles in the legs don't work independently. They work together with almost all the other muscles in the legs, trunk, shoulders, neck, and head, some muscles lengthening, some shortening, and some just holding on while you do an activity. Try running with a strained neck muscle and you will discover not just your leg muscles are working to run.

Consequently, while you are working on strengthening routines, you will also be working on flexibility and balance. While working on strengthening routines, you will be strengthening many muscles in your body simultaneously, not just one muscle. To have **Functional Strength**, many muscles work together in your arms, legs, and trunk to do a task successfully. Muscles in your body work as a team to do an activity.

Why Functional Routines?

Any activities involving reaching, bending, or twisting, such as making a bed, putting on socks, getting a box off a high shelf, or getting up and down from a chair or in and out of a car, are all made easier with the routines in this book. This is because these routines address functional strength, functional flexibility, and functional balance. **Balance, Flexibility**, and **Strength** are all required for stability, the ability to not fall down during any daily activities.

Activating the specialized mechanisms for better balance, maintaining or improving flexibility, and having functional strength keep us from getting injured in day-to-day activities or sports, and improve our sense of well-being and quality of life.

Studies show that people with a fitness routine in their life sleep better, have fewer experiences of depression, experience fewer aches and pain, have less fear of falling, and have more energy and a greater sense of well-being. Having a fitness routine leads to a better quality of life in general.

A Word About Your Brain

The brain plays a part in how well we are able to function in life. The brain knows nothing of individual muscles, ligaments, or joints. The brain knows movement patterns, such as how to get up out of a chair and walk, run, hit a golf ball, or ski. The movement routines in this book train the brain without your having to think about muscles, ligaments, or joints. Most of the routines in this book are done with one or both feet on the ground, controlling our center of gravity and contributing to stability so as not to fall down. They blend turning motion, forward and backward motion, and side-to-side motion, as well as varying speed, as these are the demands made on us in our day-to-day life activities and sports.

What you think plays a part in your success. "If you think you can do it, you can. If you think you can't do it, you can't." If you think you can get stronger, have more flexibility, and have better balance, you will be more successful in achieving improvement. If you think you can't, you may be in jeopardy of not continuing to do the functional routines for **Balance, Flexibility**, and **Strength**. Enjoy the rewards of "I can do this!"

We are only as strong as we are flexible and able to balance.

A Word About Posture

Good posture while sitting or standing or walking, makes you feel more confident and look more confident, gives you more energy, and puts less wear and tear on muscles, ligaments, and joints. Attention to good posture while sitting, standing, and walking contributes to less pain, better lung capacity, and better health in general.

There are three curves in your spine. Too much bend or too little bend in any of these curves contributes to poorer posture and a wide range of symptoms detrimental for good health.

The biggest culprits for poor posture are looking down at your cell phone while sitting, standing, or walking, and sitting at a computer for long periods of time without paying attention to your posture.

Stand tall. Think tall. Shoulders down and back. Chin tucked. Squeeze your butt. Tense your tummy. Good posture promotes a sense of well being, positively impacting our physical and emotional health. Good posture sends a body language message to others of self-confidence. Good posture is a habit. Remind yourself to have good posture while sitting, standing, or walking for a month. In the second month, recognize when you have good posture.

By the third month, good posture will be automatic. Don't forget to get up from a desk or sofa and walk around every hour and think about your good posture. Now add a long stride when you walk. Reach out to the next step heel first. Look up at where you are going, not down at a phone. Think: Stand tall. Shoulders back and down.

A Word About Toes

Why talk about toes and feet? Our feet and toes respond as soon as we want to get up and move. Feet and toes are the base of our support. Get a painful blister on your foot and see how difficult it makes walking, running, or playing a sport. But what do we do to our feet at an early age? We encase them in shoes as toddlers. Our sturdy or "supportive" shoes limit the movement of foot bones and toes that play a part in our ability to balance and not fall down. Look at your bare feet when you are sitting or standing. Can you spread your toes apart? Can you raise your toes up? Curl them down? Can you make a more prominent arch in your foot? Flatten your foot? The more we challenge our feet to support us when we move, the stronger all the little muscles in our feet get and the better they respond to help us to not fall down even when encased in shoes. So I recommend you do the routines in this book with bare feet. Then, all the little foot and toe muscles learn to respond to movement and learn to be part of the balance solution that keeps us from falling down.

CHAPTER 6

ROUTINES FOR BALANCE, FLEXIBILITY, AND STRENGTH

All routines are easier with shoes on and more challenging with shoes off, easier on a hard floor and more challenging on carpet.

A. WAKE UP YOUR BRAIN

Routines to integrate the left and right sides of your brain. Improves balance, vision, mental acuity, and ability to focus.

1. Cross Crawls: Hand to Shoulder

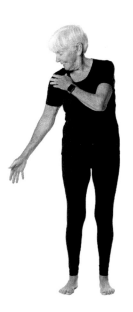

- Stand on both feet.
- Touch left hand to right shoulder and look at left hand.
- Touch right hand to left shoulder and look at right hand.
- Alternate touching and looking at your shoulders.

5 - 10 repetitions

2. Cross Crawls: Hand to Hip

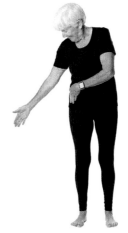

- Stand on both feet.
- Touch left hand to right hip and look at left hand.
- Touch right hand to left hip and look at right hand.
- Alternate touching and looking at your hips.

5 - 10 repetitions

3. Cross Crawls: Hand to Knees

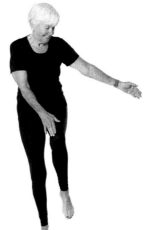

- Stand on right foot.
- Bring left knee up.
- Touch right hand to left knee.
- Look at your right hand.
- Alternate touching each knee, looking at the hand and knee touched.

5 - 10 repetitions

4. Cross Crawls: Hand to Foot

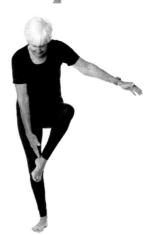

- Stand on right foot.
- Bring left knee up.
- Touch right hand to left foot.
- Look at your right hand.
- Alternate touching each foot, looking at the hand and foot touched.
- Repeat, moving free leg to the left then right across the front of your body.

5 - 10 repetitions

5. Elephant Trunk

Figure "8"

- Stand with your feet shoulder width apart.
- Clasp hands with overlapped thumbs and raise arms straight in front of you.
- Draw a figure "8" as large as you can without moving your head.
- Follow thumbs with your eyes (keep your head still).
- Go in the opposite direction.
- Can you go higher then lower while still following thumbs with just your eyes?

Side-Lying Figure "8"

- Stand with your feet shoulder width apart.
- Clasp hands with overlapped thumbs, and raise arms straight in front of you.
- Draw a side-lying figure "8" as large as you can without moving your head.
- Follow thumbs with your eyes (keep your head still).
- Then, go the opposite direction.
- Can you go farther out to each side while following thumbs with your eyes?

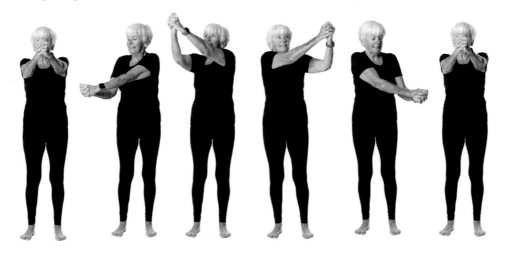

What's Working: Eye muscles improve vision and help integrate the left and right sides of your brain, contributing to a better ability to balance during activity.

B. WARM-UPS: YES? NO?

Here are some questions:

- Should you warm up your body before workout routines? No warm-up?
- Should you stretch before a workout routine? After a workout routine? Or both?

There is research that will support any of these scenarios.

I always start my workout routines by warming up my body, getting the blood flowing, and "oiling the hinges" (getting the fluid in the joints moving). I recommend you do the same.

How much time should you spend to warm-up?

Start slowly: 2-4 minutes. Gradually increase your time to achieve your personal warm-up time goal.

The goal is to get your blood moving, joints "oiled" and moving easily, not to sweat and get your heart pounding!

If your goal is a cardio workout, keep your heart rate up for 20-30 minutes by increasing the speed of your warm-up activity.

Warm-up time also depends on how much time you want to exercise each session.

Remember to keep your warm-up goal achievable...Shorter is better.

Here are some suggestions for warming up:

1. Marching in Place

- Alternate raising knees, keeping knees low.
- Hands on hips, both hands toward the ceiling, return to hips.
- Both hands up to the left, then right, return to hips.
- Both hands shoulder high out to the left, return to hips, then out to the right.
- Both hands to the ceiling and back to hips.
- Both hands touch the left knee and up overhead, then touch the right knee.
- Opposite hand to opposite knee.

2. Slow Jog in Place, Raising Knees High

3. Fast Jog in Place, Raising Knees High

4. Boxing Punches

- Stand with one foot slightly ahead of the other.
- Throw punches in the air in front of you, as if you were boxing.
- Throw punches up toward the ceiling, then down toward the floor, then out to the side.

More Challenging:

- Simulate jumping rope in place.
- Do little jumps in place.
- Skip in place.
- Hop several times on one foot, then the other.
- Jump with both feet side to side.
- Jump with both feet front and back.

For all of the above, the number of repetitions is up to you, depending on time and goal. Choose what you can do easily. This is not a contest. You just want to get the blood moving. Or choose not to do warm-ups at all!

C. BALANCE ROUTINES

Do you know how well you can balance on one foot? Balance is the ability to lose your balance, and regain it without falling. Falls and fear of falling increase as we get older. Falls also contribute to significant injuries as we get older. Studies show you can improve your balance as long as you live if you do some work daily to challenge your ability to balance.

There are many components to consider about balance.

Do the "Wake Up Your Brain" routines before you do balance routines!

To start, can you stand on one foot? For how long?

Here are the questions to consider:

1. Do you think you can stand on one foot for 5-10 seconds?

- What you think you can do influences your ability to stand on one foot.
- Tell yourself: "I can stand on one foot and balance."
- Start by standing on the foot/leg you think is the stronger or more stable.

2. Are your eyes open or closed when you stand on one foot?

It's harder to balance with your eyes closed.

3. Are you looking up? Down? Left? Right? Straight ahead?

It's easier to balance on one foot with your eyes open and focused straight ahead. Your eyes play a part in your ability to balance.

4. Are you moving your arms or other leg to assist in balance? Or are you making an effort to stand still to balance one foot?

Movement of arms, legs, head, and trunk all contribute to your ability to not lose your balance. It's OK to move while balancing on one foot. This contributes to your ability not to fall when losing your balance and returning to standing.

Let's begin with a challenge to your balance (some call this a test). It is helpful to know your starting point. How many seconds can you stand on one foot and balance without touching your hand or foot to a counter or wall for support?

Start by standing near a counter or wall that you could use to help keep your balance.

Can you stand on one foot without holding on to or touching anything? If not, can you stand on one foot using only one hand, lightly touching a counter, chair, or wall for support? If the answer is still no, can you stand on one foot using both hands lightly touching a counter?

Now see how well you are able to balance on the other foot.

Do you have the same need for support, or do you need more or less support when you stand on the other foot? It is not unusual to have better balance on one foot than on the other foot.

Do the first challenge test to see what you can do. Remember to test each leg.

Remember this journey to be fit or stay fit, and to be able to move and not fall down. It begins with accepting your **Balance**, **Flexibility**, and **Strength** where you are here and now.

Challenge Test for Balance

Clock or watch with a second hand

Date: _____

Time the number of seconds you can stand and balance with eyes open, and note if you need to lightly touch the wall or counter to stay balanced.
Left foot: _____ secs/min. Right foot: _____ secs/min

Wall, counter, or back of a chair for assist: yes: _____ no: _____

Goal 1:

- Balance on one foot without touching a counter or wall for support.

Goal 2:

- Increase the time you can balance on one foot without an assist.

Retest as often as you want to gauge your progress.

The ability to physically balance challenges many aspects of function: physical function and mental function, as in the ability to focus/concentrate on a project, and contributes to integrating the left and right sides of the brain. Balance routines support mental and emotional focus, clearing the mind to be fully present for the immediate task. Remember to breathe!

BALANCE ROUTINES

Do the Wake Up Your Brain routines first!

1. Standing Balance: One Leg

- Stand on one foot near a counter or wall for possible support.
- Use your arms or other leg to help you balance.
- Focus on a spot with your eyes open.
- Use the back of a chair, or touch a wall or counter for assistance, if necessary.
- Toe touch with the opposite foot for an assist, if necessary.

Repeat 2 to 5 times on each leg, a minimum of once a day. Shoes on is easier, shoes off is harder. Hard or wood floors are easier, and carpet is harder.

Goals:

- No chair, counter, wall, or toe touch for assistance.

2. Standing Balance: Arms Forward and Back

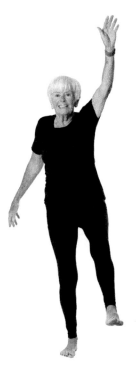

- Stand on one foot.
- Look straight ahead and focus on an object at eye level.
- Swing one arm forward and one arm back.
- Gradually increase the number of swings and keep your balance.

Variations:

- Swing fast.
- Swing slowly.
- Swing free leg forward and back.

3. Standing Balance: Eyes Moving

- Stand on one leg.
- Use arms and free leg to help you balance.
- Look up and down with just your eyes while balancing.
- Look up and down with your eyes and your head while balancing.
- Look to the left, then to the right with eyes only while balancing.
- Look left and then right, turning your head and eyes.
- Look up to the left and down to the right with your eyes only, and balance. Then switch directions.
- Look up to the left and down to the right with your eyes and head. Then switch directions.

4. Standing Balance: Arms Left and Right

- Stand on one leg.
- Move both arms to the left, then to the right.

Easier: Look straight ahead and focus on an object at eye level.

More Challenging: Look at your arms as they go to the left and right.

Variation: Move free leg side to side across the front of your body.

Goal:

- Increase repetitions

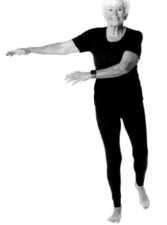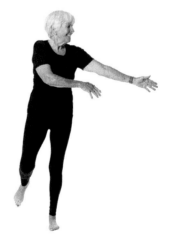

Smile! Breathe!

Summary for Balance Routines

Wake Up Your Brain

1. Cross Crawls

- Alternate touching opposite hand to opposite shoulder, hips, knees, and feet.
- Look at your hand while touching each area.

2. Elephant Trunk

- Clasp hands, look at thumb nails, make figure 8s.

Balance Routines

1. Standing Balance: One Leg

2. Standing Balance: Arms Forward and Back

3. Standing Balance: Eyes Moving, Side to Side, Up and Down

4. Standing Balance: Arms Left and Right

- Variation: Move Free Leg Side to Side Across Front of Body

Remember to repeat with the other leg.

Goals:

- No assistance with opposite toe touch or finger touch on wall or counter. Increase the time you can balance on each leg.

Smile! Breathe!

D. FLEXIBILITY ROUTINES

Upper Body Flexibility Routines

Flexibility refers to how well you are able to straighten, bend, and move. The following are flexibility routines for fingers, wrists, shoulders, neck, mid and low back, hips, feet, and eye muscles. I suggest doing these stretches with bare feet. Flexibility contributes to balance, which, in turn, contributes to stability so you don't fall down.

1. Hip Circles

- Stand with your feet shoulder width apart and hands on your hips.
- Make circles with your hips going clockwise.
- Make circles with your hips going counterclockwise.
- Stand with your feet together and hands on your hips.
- Circle hips clockwise.
- Circle hips counterclockwise.

5 - 10 Repetitions

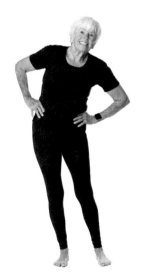 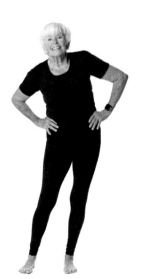 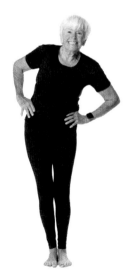

2. Clasped Fingers Overhead Reach

- Stand with your feet shoulder width apart.
- Clasp your fingers together and turn your palms down.
- Stretch your arms out in front of you and up over your head.
- Turn your body and head to the right, looking past your arm.
- Then look up with your head and eyes; look down with your head and eyes.
- Staying turned right, look left.
- Look past your left shoulder with the head and eyes; look up, look down.
- Allow your feet and ankles to roll as you turn to look past your shoulder.
- Repeat, turning to the left and looking past your arm, then turning your head and eyes to look left, then look up and down.
- Staying turned to the left, turn and look past your right shoulder and look up and down.

3 - 5 Repetitions

More challenging :

- Do the above exercise first standing on the left leg, then on the right leg.

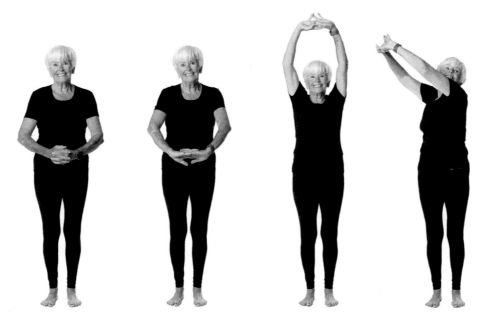

3. Crossed Arms Overhead Reach

- Stand with your feet shoulder width apart.
- Start with your arms at your sides.
- Bring your arms together in front of your body and cross your arms.
- With crossed arms, put your palms together.
- Keeping your arms straight, raise them over your head, keeping your palms together.
- Turn your body and head and look over your shoulder, past your arm.
- Holding that position, look up with your head and eyes, then look down several times.
- Repeat to the other side.

3 - 6 Repetitions

More challenging:

- Do the above exercise first standing on the left leg, then on the right leg.

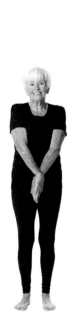 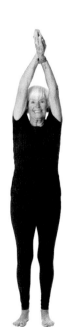 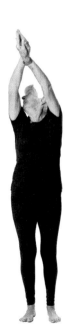 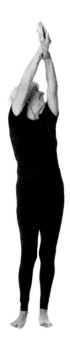

4. Shoulder/Chest Stretch With Hands Behind Your Back, Palms Down

- Stand with your feet shoulder width apart.
- Clasp your hands behind your back.
- Turn palms down.
- Slide your clasped hands up your back and down several times.
- Lift your hands away from your back and return them several times.
- Keeping your hands clasped and palms down behind your back, turn your body and head, and look over your shoulder. Your feet and ankles may roll slightly as you turn.
- Using your head and eyes, look up and down several times.
- Repeat to the opposite side.
- Remember to breathe.

3 - 6 Repetitions

More challenging:

- Do the above exercise first standing on the left leg, then on the right leg.

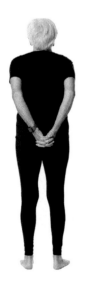 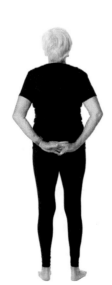 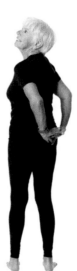 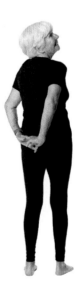

5. Shoulder/Chest Stretch Wrist Pull

- Stand with feet shoulder width apart.
- Grasp one wrist with the opposite hand behind your back.
- Gently pull that arm across your body.
- Tip your head to the side on which you are pulling your arm.
- While tipped to the side, look up to the ceiling, then down to the floor.
- Go slowly.
- Repeat to the opposite side.

3 - 6 Repetitions

More challenging:

- Do the above exercise first standing on the left leg, then on the right leg.

Smile! Breathe!

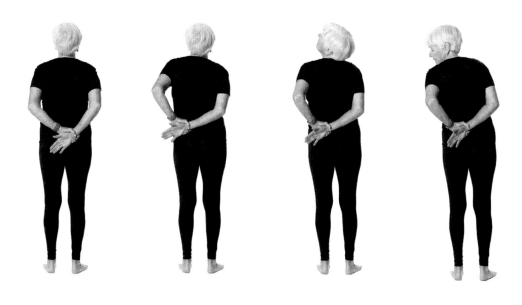

6. Full-Body Standing Stretch

- Stand with feet shoulder width apart.
- Reach up with one hand and reach down with the other.
- Bending at the waist, tip the whole body toward the hand that is down.
- Staying tipped to that side, turn your head toward the "down" hand.
- Look down and over that shoulder.
- Staying tipped, look up at the hand overhead.
- Repeat looking up and down several times.
- Staying tipped, turn your head and look under the opposite armpit.
- Remember to look with your eyes as well as with your head.
- Repeat to the other side.

3 - 6 Repetitions

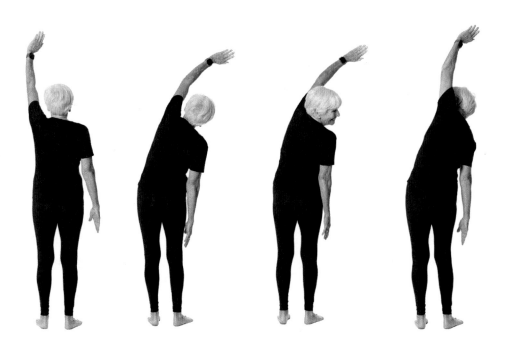

Smile! Breathe!

7. Leaves on the Trees, Fish in the Sea

1. Standing on Both Feet With One Arm Raised

- Raise your right arm out in front of you, palm down at shoulder level.
- Trace a large, side-lying "figure 8" in the air in front of you, thumb first, and allow your palm to face up, then down as you go.
- Watch your thumb using your head and eyes to follow the "8."
- Slowly make the "side-lying 8" go higher in the air and farther out to each side.
- Allow your body to turn as you go out to the sides.
- Now, in the opposite direction, trace a large, "side-lying figure 8" in the air in front of you, little finger first, and allow your palm to face up, then down, as you go.

Variations:

- "Leaves on the Trees, Swaying in the Breeze." Wiggle your fingers while making your "8" going higher.
- Slowly bring the "side-lying 8" back down below your waist, always pointing your thumb in the direction in which you make the "8" and looking at your thumb with your head and eyes.
- "Fish Swimming in the Sea." Wiggle your fingers while making your "side-lying 8" going lower. Go in the opposite direction, using your little finger as a pointer.
- Repeat with the other arm. Try on one foot.

Leaves on the Trees, Fish in the Sea (continued)

2. Standing on Both Feet, Both Arms Raised

- Big-time "Wake Up Your Brain": Make 8s with both arms.
- Extend both arms in front of you, shoulder width apart.
- Use your thumbs as pointers, left hand palm up, right hand palm down.
- Watch your hands while making the "side-lying 8s."
- Slowly go higher and higher, then lower and lower.
- Wiggle your fingers for leaves in the trees, arms going higher, and fish in the sea, arms going lower.
- Now go in the opposite direction, little fingers going first.

What's Working: Improves ability to **Balance**, shoulder and trunk **Flexibility**, and **Strength**, including eye muscles, integrating the left and right side of your brain and contributing to focus and stability.

Summary of Upper Body Flexibility Routines

1. Hip Circles

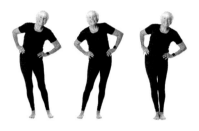

2. Overhead Reach

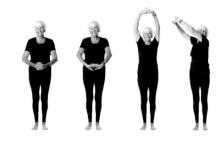

3. Straight Arms Cross

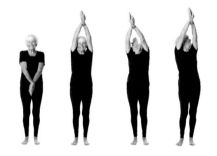

4. Clasped Hands Behind Back

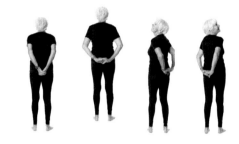

5. Clasp Opposite Wrist

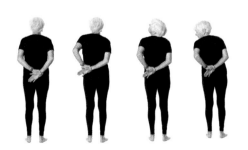

6. Full-Body Standing Stretch

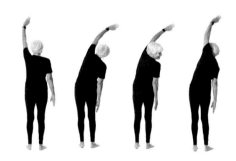

7. Leaves on the Trees, Fish in the Sea
See page 39.

Lower Body Flexibility Routines

Why be concerned about lower body flexibility? It makes it easier to get dressed, get up and down from a chair or toilet, and to get up from the floor if you fall. It also contributes to better posture for sitting, standing, and walking, with more energy in general, and keeps you feeling and looking better.

1. Bent Knee Trunk Rotation

- Lying on your back, tuck your chin, putting the back of your head on the floor.
- Bring both knees toward your chest. Hold knees with both hands if needed.
- You may have to bring one knee at a time toward your chest.
- Gently roll both bent knees to one side and toward the floor.
- Reach your arms out to the side.
- Look to the opposite side of the bent knees.
- Repeat to the other side.
- Go slowly.
- To increase the stretch, with both knees to one side, slowly straighten the top leg and lower it toward the floor.
- Repeat to the other side.

5 - 10 Repetitions

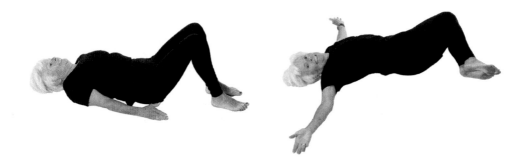

Smile! Breathe!

2. Knee to Chest Hip Stretch

- Lie on your back on the floor, knees bent, feet on the floor.
- Tuck your chin, resting the back of your head on the floor.
- Bring one knee to your chest.
- Hold the bent knee with your hands, bringing your knee closer to your chest.
- Slowly straighten the other leg, pressing that knee toward the floor.
- Release that knee, then press it toward the floor again.
- Do several press and release while continuing to hold the other knee toward your chest.
- Repeat on the opposite side.

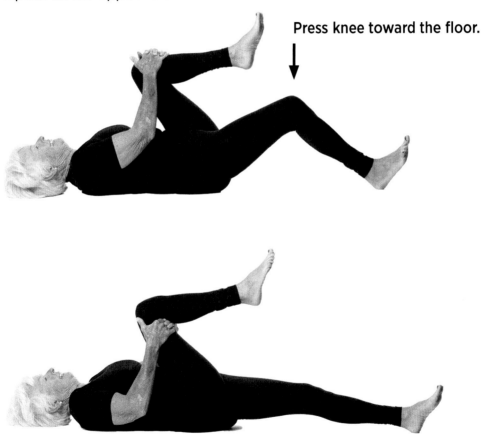

Press knee toward the floor.

3. Hamstring Flexibility

- Lie on the floor next to an open door, with both legs extended through the doorway.
- Place one leg on the doorjamb.
- Your other leg remains on the floor extended through the doorway.
- Slide the heel of the leg on the doorjamb up the wall.
- Slowly, gently press your knee toward the wall.
- Scoot your buttocks toward the wall to get more stretch in the leg on the doorjamb.
- Holding the straight leg against the doorjamb:
    - Point your toes toward the ceiling, then toward your face.
    - Point toes to the left, then to the right.
- Stay in the stretch for 1-2 minutes before sliding that leg back to the floor.
- Repeat several times.
- Repeat with the other leg.

Smile! Breathe!

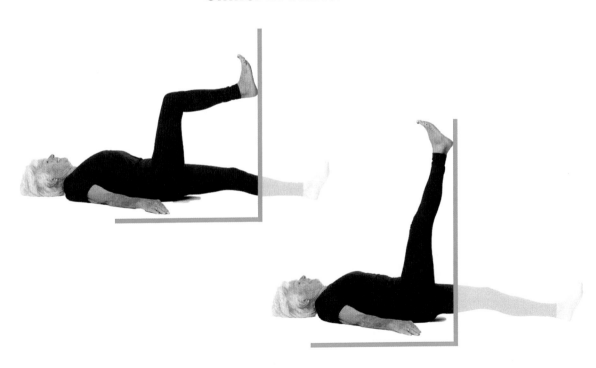

4. Alternative Hamstring Flexibility

This can be done on the floor or on a firm bed.

- Lie on your back, knees bent.
- Tuck your chin.
- Press the back of your head to the floor.
- Hold behind one knee and bring that leg toward your chest.
- Slowly straighten that leg toward the ceiling.
- Slowly straighten the other leg toward the floor.
- Press that knee toward the floor.
- Point and flex the toes of both feet, 3-6 times.
- Make ankle circles with both feet, 3-6 times.
- Continue to keep the leg on the floor as straight as possible.

Smile! Breathe!

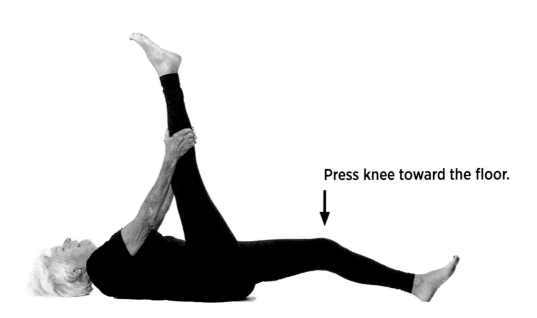

Press knee toward the floor.

5. Press Up to Back Extension

- Lie on your stomach, hands at shoulder level.
- Push up onto resting on your elbows, leaving your hips on the floor.
- Look up to the left, then look up to the right.
- Harder: Press up until your arms are straight.
- Look up to the left, then look up to the right several times.
- Return chest to the floor. Repeat 4-8 times.
- Only lift up to the point of a mild stretch, without pain.

Smile! Breathe!

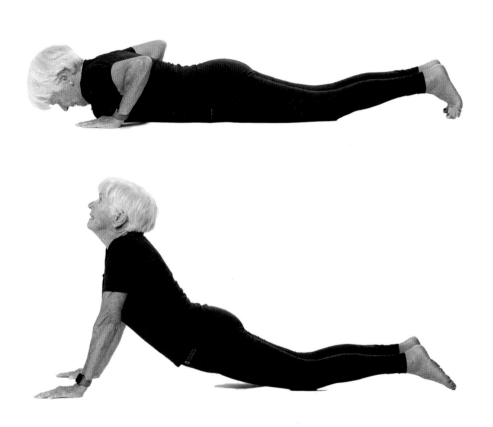

6. Hands and Knees Sit Back

- Start on your hands and knees.
- Press your "butt" back toward your feet.
- Lower head and shoulders toward the floor.
- Go only as far back as the bend in your knees allows.
- Breathe in and out slowly several times.

While rocked back, walk your hands to the left and then to the right.

Smile! Breathe!

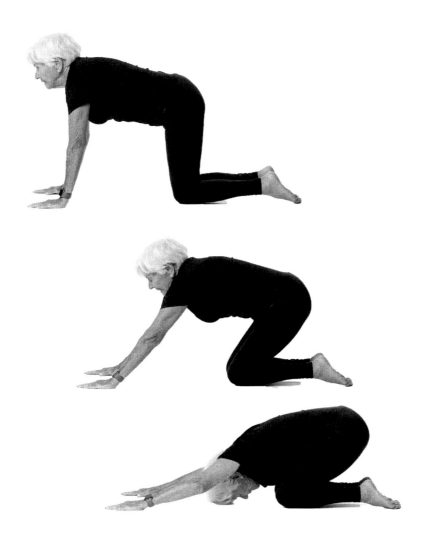

7. Full-Body Stretch and Breathe

- Lie on your back, face up.
- Extend your legs out straight.
- Take a long, slow breath in as you reach up and overhead with your arms.
- Point your toes, stretching your legs out long.
- Stretch, stretch, stretch as you breathe in.
- Release as you breathe out, letting everything go and, return your arms back to your sides.
- I like to breathe in through my nose and out through gently pursed lips.
- Stretch again, reaching up, breathing in, with toes pointed.
- I like to visualize the air going in all the way down into my toes.
- Release as you breathe out, letting everything go and, return your arms back to your sides.
- Repeat several times; go slowly.
- Lie relaxed for several minutes, breathing in and out slowly, mentally letting go of any muscle or mental tension with every breath out.

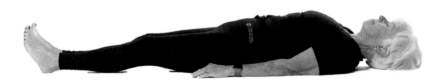

Smile! Breathe!

8. Seated Hip Stretch

"Putting on your socks" routine: neck and back flexibility.

- Sit on the edge of a chair or bench.
- Put the ankle of your right foot on your left knee.
- Hold your foot on your knee with your right hand.
- This may be as much as you can do, and that is OK.
- Breathe in and out while holding for several breaths.
- Turning your head and shoulders, look right, then look up and down several times.
- Slowly turn and look left, then look up and down several times.

To increase the stretch:

- Reach forward with your left hand resting on or below your left knee.
- Slowly slide your left hand down your shin toward the floor, only as far as you are comfortably able to do.
- Turning your head and shoulders, look right, then look up and look down.
- Slowly turn and look left, then look up and down.
- Breathe in and out several times.
- Repeat with the other leg.

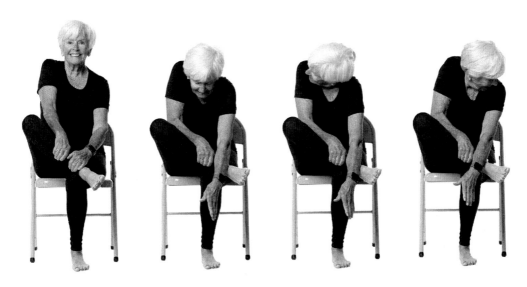

9. Static Dynamic Calf Flexibility

Review of Static and Dynamic Stretching

A static stretch is when you hold a certain position to stretch muscles and ligaments around a joint or joints to get or keep muscle length around that joint or joints. A static stretch is a non-functional stretch. A static stretch is in only one plane of motion. Our bodies move in two or three planes of motion (forward and back, side to side, turning/rotating) to do the activities of living life. We need functional muscle length and functional flexibility to get in and out of a car, bend over to pick something up off the floor, or put a cereal box on a high shelf, and during many sports activities.

A dynamic stretch is when you add movement on a static stretch. The added movement to a static stretch makes a more functional stretch. The added muscle length, around a joint or joints, helps with day-to-day activities and sports, as it incorporates two or three planes of motion.

Calf Flexibility

There are two muscles in the calf. One crosses the ankle at the back of the heel and attaches about 2/3 up the lower leg bone, the tibia. This is the soleus muscle. The soleus is a deeper muscle. The other muscle crosses the ankle at the back of the heel and crosses the back of the knee and is called the gastrocnemius muscle, or gastroc. It's a bigger muscle easily seen on the back of your lower leg. If you injure (strain) your calf muscle(s) or they become weak, you lose stability in your knee joint. If these muscles are injured, your knee feels like it will buckle and/or hyperextend. Because of the role these muscles play in the knee's stability, it is very important to keep them stretched as well as strong. Tight calf muscles can contribute to foot pain, balance issues, or knee pain. Tight (short) calf muscles are more subject to injury/strains.

Calf Flexibility Routines

There are two calf muscles to stretch, the gastroc and the soleus.
To stretch the gastroc, keep the back leg straight.
To stretch the soleus, keep the back leg bent.

1. Standing Calf Stretch: Back Leg Straight for Gastroc Stretch

- Place one foot forward and one foot back.
- Point your toes straight ahead.
- Keep your back heel on the floor, knee straight, front knee bent.
- Press hips/pelvis forward gently to increase the stretch. Stand tall.
- While holding the stretch, slowly reach around with both hands to the left.
- Turn your head and shoulders to look around to the left and behind you.
- Repeat, turning around to the right.
- Get a sense of where the most tension develops in the calf muscle.
- Hold there, breathing in and out several times slowly.
- Then continue turning left and right.
- Remember to keep the toes on both feet pointing straight ahead.

2. Standing Calf Stretch: Back Knee Bent for Soleus Stretch

- Follow the previous directions, but with a slight bend in the back knee.
- Keep your heel on the floor.

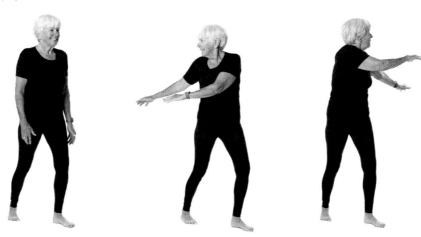

Variations:

- Turn both feet about 45 degrees to the left and repeat the above routine.
- Turn both feet to the right about 45 degrees and repeat the above routine.

3. Standing Gastroc Calf Stretch

Using a wall or counter.

- Stand facing a wall or counter, about 8-12 inches away.
- Put your hands against the wall or counter.
- Take a step back with one foot.
- Point your toes straight ahead.
- Bend the knee on the front leg.
- Looking straight ahead, move your hips toward the wall/counter until you feel a stretch in the calf of the back leg.
- Keep your back heel on the floor and knee straight.
- Bending at the elbows, lean forward, keeping your hands on the wall or counter, and do several press-ups against the wall/counter.
- Press hips/pelvis forward gently while doing the press-ups.
- Look up while doing the stretch with press-ups.
- Reach around to the right, looking at your hand with your head and eyes.
- While turned, look up and then down several times.
- Repeat, turning to the left.

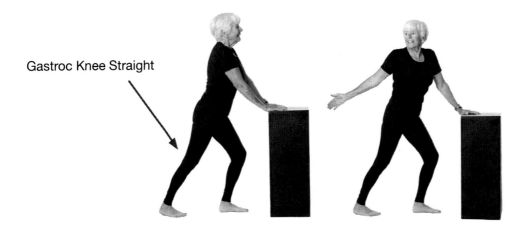

Gastroc Knee Straight

4. Standing Soleus Calf Stretch

Using a wall or counter.

- Stand facing a wall or counter, about 8-12 inches away.
- Place hands on the wall or counter.
- Take a step back with one foot, about 6-10 inches.
- Keep both feet facing forward. Look forward.
- Slightly bend **BOTH** knees.
- Move your chest toward the wall/counter until you feel a stretch in the calf of the back leg.
- Keep both heels on the floor, feet facing forward.
- Reach around to the right, looking at your hand with your head and eyes.
- While turned, look up and then down several times.
- Repeat, turning to the left.

Variations:

- Turn both feet about 45 degrees to the left and repeat the above routine.
- Then turn both feet to the right about 45 degrees and repeat the above routine.

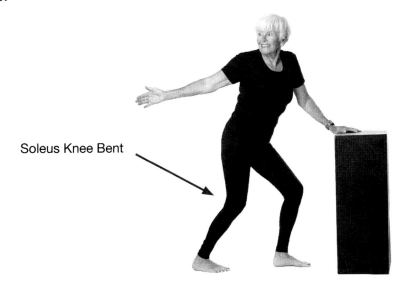

Soleus Knee Bent

Summary of Lower Body Flexibility Routines

1. Bent Knee Trunk Rotation

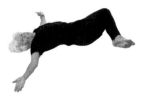

2. Knee to Chest Hip Stretch

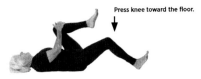

Press knee toward the floor.

3. Hamstring Flexibility

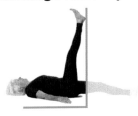

4. Alternative Hamstring Flexibility

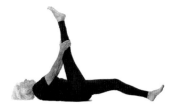

5. Press Up to Back Extension

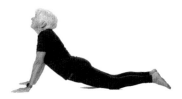

6. Hands and Knees Sit Back

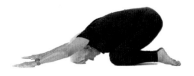

7. Full-Body Stretch and Breathe

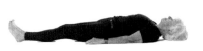

8. Seated Hip Stretch

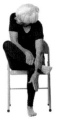

9. Calf Flexibility Routines

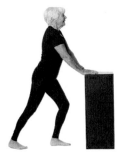

"The most important thing to remember is this: to be ready at any moment to give up what you are for what you might become."

- W. E. B. Du Bois, scholar and activist

"It is not the strongest of the species that survives, nor the most intelligent, but the one most responsive to change."

- Charles Darwin, biologist, 1809-1882

*"If you are the 'pilot' of your life, who needs a runway?
Take off right where you are!"*

- Vernice "Fly Girl" Armour was the first female African-American naval aviator in the United States Marine Corps and combat pilot flying SuperCobra attack helicopters

Smile! Breathe!

E. STRENGTH ROUTINES

Calf Strengthening: Toe Raises

The flexibility and strength of calf muscles contribute to knee stability. Knee stability refers to knees that don't feel like they will buckle or hyper-extend, causing you to lose balance or fall. Calf muscle strength contributes to overall balance and stability.

First, can you stand on one foot and raise up onto your toes, with or without touching a counter or wall for support? If you cannot do one or two toe raises on one foot, do the challenge test and the exercise standing on both feet. It's easier with shoes on and harder without shoes.

CHALLENGE TESTS FOR CALF STRENGTH

1. Standing on Both Legs
Toe Raises to Measure Calf Strength

If you cannot stand on one foot and do toe raises, do them standing on both feet. How many can you do on both feet before you can't do them anymore?

Stop if you have pain, or do fewer, or don't raise up as high onto your toes.

Date of Test: _____   # Reps: _____

Goal:

To do toe raises standing on one foot with or without touching a wall or counter for balance.

2. Standing on One Leg
Single-Leg Toe Raises to Measure Calf Strength

Stand on one foot, with or without touching a counter or wall for balance, and raise yourself up and down onto the ball of your foot.

How many toe raises (lifting your heel off the floor to stand on forefoot and toes) can you do?

How many can you do on the left foot? How many on the right foot? Do you need to touch a wall or counter for balance? Do not use the wall or counter to help you raise up onto your toes. Just use it to keep your balance.

Moving your arms or legs for balance is OK.

Date of Test:_____

Reps Left: _____   Balance Assist: Yes: _____   No:_____

Reps Right:_____   Balance Assist: Yes: _____   No:_____

STRENGTHENING ROUTINES

1. Calf Strengthening Toe Raises: Standing on Both Feet

- How many toe raises could you do on challenge test #1?
- For the strengthening routine, do 3-5 fewer.
- You can choose whether or not you want to repeat this after a brief rest. Remember, less is better.
- Smile and breathe!

Goal:

Be able to do single-leg toe raises and increase repetitions.

2. Calf Strengthening Toe Raises: Standing on One Foot

- If you need to touch a wall or furniture or touch a toe to the ground for balance, do so.
- If you can you do more repetitions if you touch a wall or counter to balance, then do it!
- Stand on one foot. Slightly bend the leg you're standing on.. Lift your heel off the floor as you rise up to stand on your forefoot and toes, then put your heel back down.
- Start with 5-10 repetitions.
- Stop when or if it becomes difficult or painful.
- Do one leg, then the other. The number of reps on each leg may vary.

Your arms or other leg may move around to help you balance while doing the toe raises. Balance is the ability to recover as you sway/move in and out of being balanced. Balance is not about standing still.

Moving arms or the other leg for balance is OK.

Variations for 1 and 2:

- Go very fast. Go very slowly.
- Look to the left, eyes open.
- Hold weights or soup cans!
- Look to the right, eyes open;
- Close your eyes: go fast; go slowly.

Goal:

To not use your hands on the wall, furniture, or touch a toe to the ground to assist with balance. Increase number of repetitions as you're able.

What's Working: Calf muscles, foot, ankle, thigh (quadriceps and hamstrings), butt, abdominal and back muscles, and improves balance and stability!

Smile! Breathe!

Standing Balance Reach...
Sneaking in Flexibility and Strength

3. Standing Balance Reach: Standing on both feet
(Easiest)

- Stand on both feet about 18 to 30 inches away from a wall.
- Keep your feet/toes facing forward toward the wall and not at an angle.
- Place a hand on a chair, counter, or wall next to you to assist, if needed.
- Bending at the hips, knees, and ankles, reach one hand toward the wall. Touch the wall.
- Slide your hand down as far as is comfortable and pain-free.
- Return to standing.
- Reach that arm up toward the ceiling. Stand up tall.
- If you can touch the floor and return to standing, step back a few inches until you can't go all the way to the floor and return to standing.
- Place a sticky note or tape on the wall where you touched the wall and return to standing.
- Place a sticky or tape on the floor to mark the front of your toes.
- Put a second sticky or tape 3-5 inches above the first wall sticky.
- Stand at the tape on the floor and reach the new, higher-wall sticky 4-5, times.
- Return to standing between each reach and raise that arm over your head.
- If you have pain, don't go as low on the wall. You don't want any pain.
- Alternate arms reaching to the sticky on the wall and returning to standing, then reaching that arm to the ceiling and standing tall.
- Alternate feet and repeat 3 to 5 times.

More Challenging:

- Increase the number of repetitions.
- Lower the upper sticky 1-3 inches.
- Turn your feet 45 degrees to the left and reach to touch the wall.
- Turn your feet 45 degrees to the right and reach to touch the wall
- Hold a weight or soup can and reach to touch the wall.

Goal:

- Not to touch counter or wall for assistance.

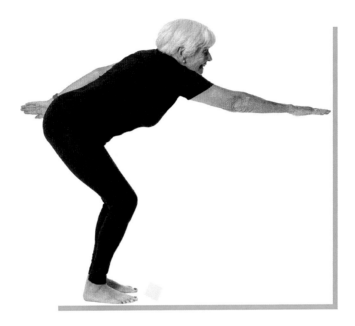

Bending at the hips, knees, and ankles, reach one hand toward the wall. Touch the wall.

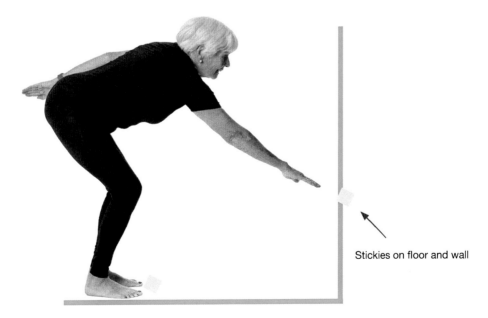

Stickies on floor and wall

Slide your hand down as far as is comfortable and pain-free.

4. Single-Leg Balance Reach
(More Challenging)

Stand on one leg, balance, reach toward the wall

- Keep your foot facing forward toward the wall and not at an angle.
- If you are unable to stand on one leg to balance, use a chair or wall for light assistance.
- Bending at the hip, knee, and ankle, reach one hand toward the wall, and touch the wall as far down as you can, pain-free!
- Return to standing.
- Lift that arm toward the ceiling, standing up tall.
- If you can touch the floor and return to standing, step back a few inches until you can't go all the way to the floor and return to standing.
- Place a sticky note at the point on the wall you can touch and on the floor in front of your toes.
- Put a second sticky or tape 2-3 inches above the first sticky.
- Stand at the sticky on the floor and reach the new wall sticky 4 -5 times, returning to standing between each reach.
- Alternate arms reaching to sticky on the wall and returning to standing, reaching that arm to the ceiling and standing tall.
- Repeat, alternating legs, 3 - 5 repetitions on each foot and alternate hand touching the wall.

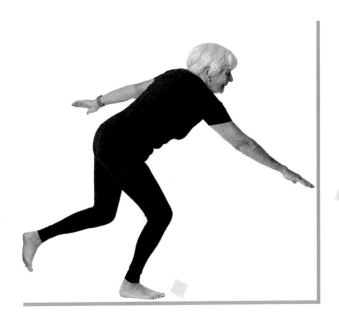

Stickies on floor and wall

Single-Leg Balance Reach Variations:

- Increase the number of repetitions.
- Lower the upper sticky 1-3 inches.
- Turn your foot 45 degrees in and reach, alternating hands.
- Return to standing and reaching that arm toward the ceiling. 4-10 repetitions.
- Turn your foot out 45 degrees and reach, alternating hands.
- Return to standing and reaching that arm toward the ceiling. 4-10 repetitions.
- Repeat with the other foot.
- Hold a 2- or 3-pound weight or a soup can to reach toward the wall and return to standing.

Goal:

Not touching the counter or wall or toe to the floor for support.

What's Working: All foot, ankle, leg, hip and trunk, stomach, and back muscles are working, getting stronger while improving flexibility and balance to increase stability.

This is a great "butt" strengthener/toner!

This routine is the secret sauce for improving Balance, Flexibility, and Strength in one routine!

Smile! Breathe!

5. Wall or Counter Push-Ups

- Stand on two feet about 18-24 inches from a wall or counter.
- Place both hands on the wall or counter, elbows straight.
- Slowly lean into the wall, bending your elbows, and then push away back to straight elbows.

More Challenging:

- Stand on one foot about 14-18 inches from a wall or counter.
- Place your hands on the wall or counter, elbows straight.
- Lean toward the wall or counter, bending your elbows and slowly push away, back to straight elbows.

3 - 10 Repetitions, and Increase Repetitions as You Want

Smile! Breathe!

Summary of Strength Routines

1. Calf Strengthening Toe Raises: Standing on Both Feet

- Stand on both feet and raise up onto your toes, with or without touching a counter or wall.

2. Calf Strengthening Toe Raises: Standing on One Foot

- Stand on one foot and raise up onto your toes, with or without touching a counter or wall.

3. Standing Balance Reach: Standing on Both Feet

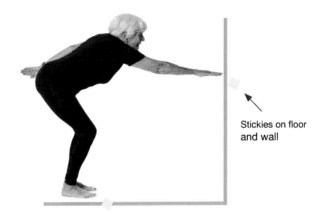

Stickies on floor and wall

4. Single-Leg Balance Reach

5. Wall or Counter Push-Ups

Smile! Breathe!

CHAPTER 7

QUALITY OF LIFE ROUTINES

A few routines to have the best quality of life as you move through life's journey.

1. Getting Down to the Floor and Up From The Floor

Why:

Many falls happen outside or on the throw rug in the middle of the house. You may ask, "If I can't get up without some assistance like a chair or sofa, do I call 911 to get help?" Only if you have your phone with you! "No, I do my **Down to the Floor and Up From the Floor** routines every day, so I know I can get up if I fall."

Requires **Balance**, **Flexibility**, and **Strength**.

Test:

- Can you get down to the floor, lie down, and get back up without assistance from furniture or walls?

The Routine:

- Get down to the floor, lie down, then get back up.
- You may do the **Lower Extremity Flexibility** routines while you are on the floor!
- Use furniture, walls, or whatever it takes to get down and back up.
- Start by doing it once a day.
- Work up to 2-3 times a day to get stronger.

Goal:
To not use any assistive devices, wall, chair, table, or sofa.

2. Sit-to-Stand Routine: Get Up and Down From the Toilet

Strengthens all leg muscles, abdominal and back muscles, and improves ability to balance.

Basic Sit-to-Stand:

- Sit on a firm chair.
- Move to the front edge of the chair.
- Lean forward, looking up as you stand up on both legs.
- While standing, move backward until the back of one or both legs touches the chair seat.
- Look up while sitting down.

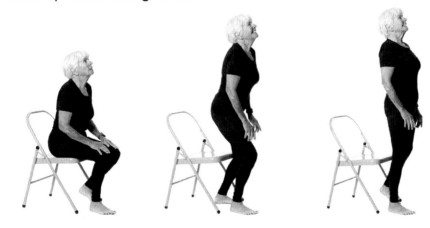

- **3 - 5 Repetitions**

Easier:
- Use a chair with arms and repeat the Basic Sit-to-Stand-to-Sit

Much Easier:
- Put one or more pillows on the chair seat and repeat the basic Sit-to-Stand

Goal:

Sit and stand without using the pillows or arms of the chair for assistance. Repeat several times until easy to do without arms or pillows on the chair. **Always look up to stand up from a chair and to sit back down in a chair.**

A Brief Talk About Posture

Good posture while sitting, standing, or walking tall makes you look and feel younger.

Good posture gives you more energy and has less wear and tear on muscles, ligaments, and joints.

- Sit tall. Stand tall. Walk tall. Think tall.
- Shoulders down and back. Chin tucked.
- Squeeze your butt. Keep tension in your tummy.
- Keep your pelvic floor muscles pulled up, in, and tight. Men and women have pelvic floor muscles.
- Step out to walk, heel first, toes up, and have a long stride.

Good posture is a habit.

Remind yourself to have good posture for a month while sitting, standing, and walking. In the second month, recognize when you have good posture or change it if you notice you are slumping.

Give yourself a little pat on the back for catching any slumping and changing it! By the third month, good posture will be automatic.

Look up to sit down in a chair; look up to stand up from a chair. It's easier to have good posture on a firm chair. Big, cushioned, comfortable chairs contribute to slumped, poor posture.

Smile! Breathe!

CHAPTER 8
SUGGESTIONS TO THINK ABOUT AND HOW TO BEGIN

I vary the routine day to day to include some balance routines, upper body or lower body flexibility, and some strengthening.

Choose just enough routines and just enough repetitions to be successful in meeting your Action Plan. Don't even think of doing all the exercises in one session. Some days, I just do upper body flexibility routines or just lower body flexibility routines, Wake Up Your Brain, and some balance routines.

If you only do 10 minutes when you have a goal of 20 minutes, don't be hard on yourself. It's ok. My goal is to do something every day. My next goal is to set an achievable amount of time, so I can continue to be successful at doing something every day. It is better to do only a few routines than to skip that day because you don't have time to meet your time goal or choices of routines for that day's goal.

When stretching and doing functional flexibility routines, go slowly. Go to the "tightness." Do not force more stretch. Don't do anything that causes pain or increases pain. Breathe while stretching!

We tend to lose **Balance**, **Flexibility**, and **Strength**, as well as good posture, as we get older. "Use it or lose it!" So my personal overall goal is to:

- Pay attention to my posture, which makes me feel and look better in general.
- Do balance exercises daily so I can recover my balance and not fall from tripping or reaching too far.
- Stretch to stay flexible so I can get in and out of my car easily.
- Stay strong so I can continue my sports activities easily.

Be aware that you may need to go to a gym or fitness center for the motivation of working out with others. For some people, going to a gym may be discouraging, watching incredibly fit folks doing way more than you can do. What motivates you?

Several routines have a test to see what you can do now. If you share the book or challenge tests with friends or spouses, please remember these are your results for where you are in the present moment. You are not having a contest with friends or a partner. You are looking to improve your results over time or maintain your fitness level. When you set a goal to improve, make it achievable. Track your improvements in a journal. Writing down your progress is motivating.

Rule: You should experience no pain when you do any of the routines. If you experience pain, don't bend as far, reach as far, or turn as far, and do fewer repetitions or skip that routine entirely for that day.

Learning styles: We all have our own learning style, which influences our ability to learn something new. Do you know what your learning style is?

- Do you like the how and why of things explained to you?
- Do you like physically doing things?
- Do you like watching something be done before doing it?
- Do you like reading a description of what to do or seeing a diagram?

Learning styles are addressed in this book, with descriptions of routines, pictures of routines, and why certain muscles are at work, or what those muscles do for your quality of life.

Energy, Enthusiasm, Healthy, Happy! I can do it!

Smile! Breathe!

Yes...you can do it!

CHAPTER 9

SUGGESTIONS FOR MAKING A FITNESS PLAN

1. Do a physical activity to get warmed up   3 - 5 Minutes

- Jogging in place (See Warm-Up Routines).
- Walking briskly outside or on a treadmill.
- Elliptical, Nordic Track, StairMaster, stationary bike.
- "Lubricates" the joints and gets the blood flowing.

2. Balance or Flexibility Routines   2 - 5 Minutes

- Wake Up Your Brain Routines.
- A Balance Routine.
- Pick 2 or 3 from the Upper Body Routines.
- Next day, pick 2 or 3 from the Lower Body Routines.
- Change the 2 or 3 routines each day.
- Remember to breathe.

3. Strength Routine

Choose one or two each day you plan your
Fitness Routines.

Change up routines each day until you have done
all routines, then start over.

- Calf Strengthening
- Balance Reach
- Sit-to-Stand Routine

4. Flexibility Routine

- Repeat the ones you started with or choose
  2-3 different Flexibility Routines.

TOTAL: 10 - 20 minutes

Smile! Breathe!

CONCLUDING WORDS

There are words and phrases in this book that came from other books, publications, and other physical therapists. They were accumulated over many years. I, in turn, shared my exercise files with fellow physical therapists. These ideas, words, and phrases became part of my mantra with my clients over 30 years and have found their way into this publication.

Today's research and publications on the role exercise plays in our day-to-day health are copious. So, I chose not to use footnotes or make a list of more current books or research that include the importance of exercise in our health and quality of life.

My goal is to keep routines easy and not to offer too many routines, so they can easily become part of your daily life.

Enjoy continuing to move through your life being fit and healthy!

Sandy Mortensen, PT

ACKNOWLEDGMENTS

I am grateful for the many people who have passed through my personal and professional lives in the last 60 years who made direct or indirect contributions to this publication.

Thank you, Mary Dahlager, Mary Headley, John Gwin, Betsy Sather, Bob Follett, Jean Curtin, James Johnson, Craig McNeil, Peter Freed, Leslie McEnary, Nell Witting, my Copper Mountain Monday ski friends, and my heli-ski friends for your contributions to and continued support to this project.

Thank you, Peter Freed, for taking the photos in this publication. I value your friendship and support for the last 44 years.

https://peterfreed.com/about

Thank you, Craig McNeil, for taking the photos in the many drafts of this publication that contributed to my completing the project and for your friendship and support for this project over the years.

https://mcneildesignerportraits.com/portraits

Thank you, James Johnson, a friend and business consultant, for your continued support to finish this project.

https://www.l3ps.com

A special thank you to my son, Zachary Mortensen, for editing, compiling, and laying out the book to get it ready for publishing. Also thank you, Zach, for your continued quiet persistence and support to get this book completed.

Many clients came through my physical therapy clinics or were seen by me in a hospital clinic. Through them, I learned about the many challenges of exercising to rehabilitate from injuries or surgeries. I appreciate their sharing their resistance to exercise and how they overcame their challenges. I appreciate their feedback on exercises. Their feedback on successes and overcoming resistance to exercise led to many revisions of this book.

In recent years, friends wanted suggestions about exercises to help with complaints of pain, weakness, and instability interfering with their quality of life. Through them, I learned to focus on the challenges of beginning a program and making exercise a daily habit. That list of friends is long and varied. Thank you for asking for help and your feedback. You helped me focus on simplicity and fewer routines that are easy to do anywhere and without equipment. You brought to my attention the importance of the voice in our heads that plays a part in successfully starting and continuing a fitness routine.

Two physical therapists influenced my professional and personal lives, and I am grateful for their seminars and friendship.

John Barnes, PT, introduced me to looking at and listening to a person's body through Myofascial Release and Cranial Sacral Therapy. Through John, I first began looking at the body as a whole entity, not just parts, and looking at restrictions to movement components and use of Myofascial Release. "Unwinding," shows up in the routine, Fish in the Sea, Leaves in the Trees.

https://www.myofascialrelease.com/about/johnfbarnes.aspx

Gary Gray, DPT, was also one of my more influential mentors. He further influenced me to look at our bodies as a whole, all parts working together in three planes of motion, feet on the ground. Through Gary's seminars, I learned more about how pain, injury, surgery, or just living on the face of the Earth can cause movement dysfunction in one area, affecting movement in other parts of our body.

I am grateful for becoming aware of the use of simple movement and strength routines in three planes of motion to regain function, not only with my clients, but to regain my shoulder function after surgical repair of all my shoulder rotator cuff tendons. This quote from the Gray Institute website says it all: "Gray Institute® exists to influence the lives of others through movement."

https://grayinstitute.com/about-us

Seminars, books, conversations with friends, and teaching childbirth classes for 14 years contributed to my awareness of the part our brain, our thoughts, and our attitudes play in the quality of our lives. Beginning or continuing a fitness program that contributes to a quality life begins with thinking positively about being fit and deciding to make changes to be fit. This also led to the awareness of how my thoughts may interfere with my quality of life in general. I slowly realized I was in charge of those thoughts. I could change my beliefs when those thoughts were not contributing to a quality life. Movement in three planes of motion, **Balance**, **Flexibility,** and **Strength** routines, are now a daily habit so I can improve my quality of life until the end of my life.

Sandy Mortensen, PT

Made in the USA
Las Vegas, NV
17 May 2025

22309143R00050